The End Is in the Middle

Also by Daniel Scott Tysdal

Poetry
Fauxccasional Poems
The Mourner's Book of Albums
Predicting the Next Big Advertising Breakthrough Using a Potentially
Dangerous Method

Fiction
Wave Forms and Doom Scrolls

Non-Fiction
The Writing Moment: A Practical Guide to Creating Poems

THE END IS IN THE MIDDLE

mad fold-in poems

DANIEL SCOTT TYSDAL

icehouse poetry
an imprint of Goose Lane Editions

Edited by Katie Fewster-Yan.
Cover and page design by Julie Scriver.
Cover illustration and author portrait by Richard Wang, instagram.com/spectre_ink.
Printed in Canada by Rapido.
10 9 8 7 6 5 4 3 2 1

Goose Lane Editions acknowledges the generous support of the Government of Canada, the Canada Council for the Arts, and the Government of New Brunswick.

Library and Archives Canada Cataloguing in Publication

Title: The end is in the middle : mad fold-in poems / Daniel Scott Tysdal.
Names: Tysdal, Daniel Scott, 1978- author.
Identifiers: Canadiana 20220192618 |
ISBN 9781773102719 (softcover)
Classification: LCC PS8639.Y84 E53 2022 |
DDC C811/.6—dc23

Goose Lane Editions is located on the unceded territory of the Wəlastəkwiyik whose ancestors along with the Mi'kmaq and Peskotomuhkati Nations signed Peace and Friendship Treaties with the British Crown in the 1700s.

Goose Lane Editions
500 Beaverbrook Court, Suite 330
Fredericton, New Brunswick
CANADA E3B 5X4

gooselane.com

once again
and always, these
rumpled poems —
each furrowed
turn and worded
fold — open through
and for

and
r
ea

Fold and live to fold again.
— The Comeback Kid

I have such a hard time accepting love.
— The Mad King

Contents

A Note on Form

The fold-in poetry form was inspired by one of my childhood heroes: Al
Jaffee. For fifty-six years, his illustrated fold-ins comprised the back inside
cover of every issue of *MAD* magazine (Jaffee retired in 2020, when he
turned 100). A page-filling image, with a brief caption at the bottom, would
be transformed by folding the page to reveal a visual and textual punchline.
Borrowing Jaffee's fold-in technique, the fold-in poem is characterized by
three features: 1) the poem does not end at the bottom of the page, 2) the
reader completes the poem by folding the page in so that the A guide meets
the B guide, and 3) these folds reveal the final line of the poem nested within
the original lines. For accessibility reasons, the final, post-fold line also
appears after each poem.

MAD
ME

A Mad Fold-In Poem

You — this mucky fire slathered in my mind's
  frame — are as committed to me as artists are
    to art. At times, your voice is constant: "Kill
   yourself, kill yourself, kill yourself" — fists
     punching clay with the aim to make me nothing
  more than punched clay. Other times,
you're a cinema in my skull, screening me
mangled: leg auger-mauled, hand
      vice-crushed, eye pencil-blinded to life —
   "End it," you say, in the scene you
     loop: this cinema's walls with a bullet
      burst. At parties, you stage a self-
    curtaining play from others' glances: "hate
him," "idiot," "fool." When I bloom, a sun,
    all alight and rising, you flatten my lift
  into lines on a page
like Jaffee's in the back of *MAD*; you fold it over
     and now the rise is the wound from a wing
  cleaved and then gilded, the sun's the mouth of
   a scum-crusted drain, the bloom's a thousand
  foot fall. Without relent, the strangling
   chorus of you circles me and sings:

You

ill

nothing

you
mangled
life —

let
self-
hate

lift

like
a wing
of
sand

~

Bubble

Kidhood is a kite's climb — you waver
                        and whip in the clouds. The wind
            pauses. You plummet. Or gales rage
against your sail and rip you loose. As a boy,
        I could fly, costumed in Supe's cape
        or squealing R2-D2's beeps with paper *Star*
        Wars cups circling X-wing flights around
        my wrists. As a boy, I could never really fly,
    skin already grounded by the shame of
        failing by living, the ball we all catch before
            it's tossed. Like the time I stole the Lego
            man from kindergarten and blamed
                my best friend. Inside me burned the cloud-
    tormenting sun that yearns to turn my soil
    to ash. Just the other day, I hated myself
        for hating myself. The shock waves
blinded every distance-binding bridge. Our
        shackles, hissing, "Stay down," constrict
                that tight. One day, I will fly. When I
            am a boy again. The kite of time
                        is a perpetual child. In its climb,
            in each second's tug, we are made
        new — returned. Sometimes, I hear
        my dad's voice. "Sonny boy," he
    says. "Sonny, it's time to get up," and
I'm a boy again. Or know that I can't be,
    but will be anyway. "Sonny," he says, and

wind

against

skin

cloud-

blinded

I

climb,

Our Kind

Marked as afflicted, we're afflicted with treatment:
whomp of lobotomy, exorcism's curse, society-
cancelling confinement, jacket-barred movement,
                    skulls drilled, temples electric, pills that sightsee
and, like brute tourists, poach horns, leave meat behind.
            We're a mouth that sears the thermometer's degrees.
            Who can cure our kind?

                Dismissed as weak, feeble shirkers, few believe
            there's victory in our loss, missing the vigour — wise
and devoted — it takes to start the car, and wait, and breathe;
            the imagination and drive required to devise
            a shotgun helmet to blast the driven, devising mind.
            We're a puzzle undone, shedding pieces like leaves.
            Who can solve our kind?

                Misjudged as fakes, we have no magic anthem
            to chant what haunts our heads into the world. What a brace
our brain is — it snaps our bones. Picture a neck as stem
            for a foul bouquet of shouting maws, skin as the base
kindling for permanent fire, guts as the food life bites and grinds.
            We're the mug they'd pummel if they could glimpse our face.

who
can
  see
and

  believe

and

  em
  brace
our

kind

Aloft

What most people don't know about barns is they're
                      playgrounds. Our fallow hayloft is home to the
shaky hoop with its awry plywood backboard I
wished for and Dad built. Great grandpa's wagon
                and the tarped grain truck are ideal trenches for toy
assault-rifle war. Most don't know barns are museums.
            The dust-mossed bone of the hammer grandpa, linnet
        frail, put down, never to lift again, is buried under the
carcasses of other unraised tools, the strata of
                    their replacements. A century of licence plates dresses
        the wall in obscure, rusting glyphs. Barns are zoos, too,
leashing cats, mice, pigeons, flies, rats, moths, foxes,
                    owls, and, when feline hunts are halted by weather,
the roadkill we drag in to feed them. What most
        don't know about barns is they're where farm boys
            tend to end it. My bus-mate, barely a teen, hung
            himself from a tie beam. After high school, an old b-ball
        pal cracked a shell in a stall. There's the end I almost
lodged into our barn's memory, another blunt tool
                    · to store in its elasticity and debris, its dusk-sifted
        palette, its age-planed wood, in the thin cylinders
            of light tunneling through slits in tin siding —
junk searchlights which the sterile pollen of dust motes
        cloud. What I don't know is if we depart for the barn
                because we're tilted goldfish drawn to the honest
rayless dark of the artificial castle, or whether,
            remarkably, vanishing from touch, we crave the weight
of the vital, janky cradles of playground, museum,
        and zoo, of hammer, fox, and hoop, a final
    grazing of the olden and acquainted that eases like

the
s
wish

as
net

car
resses

lea
ther,
the

ball

lo
fted

ju

st
r
ight

Suicide

Suicide is not an act. It's an ache
ended. A pact signed with such force
it breaks. An ace pilot kamikaze-ing
for the last cause: peace. An art apt to
deafen speaking, invisible sight. An alt-ant
that evolved from explosives — the cratered,
withering heart its hill. Suicide is a tack-
packed cat, more metal than skin, nude
and coastal with blood and yowls. Suicide is
the fact of the sealed aquarium. Inside,
the seahorse convulses, strangled by its
brother's tail. The fish's lungs collapse
from an acre to an inch. Feel that? Suicide
shatters the glass, releasing the seahorse,

end
   ing

dea
th
with
  de
a

th

Asylum Blues

Daniel doesn't know why he kept the Canon
Hi8 tapes. At twenty, he gathers and bags
them, all the flicks as a teen he shot (a synonym
in his head for "shit"). Shame's a noxious
projector lodged in his chest. It flings a stool-y,
assaulting film, un-flushing his crappy titles,
The End of Jest, Asylum Blues, Plastic Face IV, his
fermented sewage works. It's not movies but old,
dried turds he trashes in the bin behind his building;
he doesn't know what hurts worse: that he saved this
analog waste for years or failed to add more, carrion

fresh. If only he could lens himself through his
camcorder's namesake: Canon, *Guan Yin,* Goddess
of Mercy. If only he could mercy himself the lost
lightning of laughter he and his little bro flashed while
shooting the absurd *Asylum Blues,* take after cockeye
take cracking up as Nate failed to, straight-faced, ask
their prop arachnid: "Why do you mock me, spider?"
If only he grasped in glee, not pain, the ancient adage:
ars est merda, the mercy of art: "art is shit" —
fertilizing, uniting, ephemeral, necessary,
awesome in its endlessness. The spider of art
mocks us for bemoaning our web's failure to sway
in the high branches forever, forgetting impending
spinnerets will weave new strands as astonishing,
impermanent, singular, and

anon

ym
ous

as
The
ferm

ion

ca
st
light
ye

ars

aw
ay

Lift

One of the worst pains I've known is waking bloodshot
from a how-long-has-it-been bender in filthy light — misbegun
digestion souring my nostrils, blanket, lips, and
tongue — and not recognizing my face in the mirror,
or the nerves in my skin, or my brain vacated except for this
living, clamorous choice erupting across the plastered surface
of my spirit like a blister lifted by lye and more lye:
I needed to expire, or I needed to expire the bottomless
bottoming nights that ended with slurred me blearying
two triple vodka crans at last call for doubles and triples,
and two single vodka crans at last call. Drying out
doesn't refer to the lack of drink, but to the effect
this lack fractures into the molecular marrow of
me-ness: the drying out of any rivulet of sense or fable
or nectar, of any palpitating vein of the past or future or
wondrous, workaday present — the self's desiccated beds unfit
to stream anything but this pain, right now. Once, I laughed

in disbelief when the buddy I bartended with admitted he hit
a jerrycan in high school, huffing gas. He and I were killing
a dead night behind the bar by trading excess myths, a pair
of shepherds in a modern pastoral competing to see who
most stupidly stretched being's cohesion without
snapping — fifteen Gravol, a bottle of Benylin, three Everclear
shots, a pile of powdered nutmeg, eight grams of mushrooms
(half of them picked out of a girlfriend's vomit). Sobered
after his petrol confession, my buddy continued, his brio
run dry. It was on a lark at a party, this decision to huff.
Even with cases of Kokanee chilling in the fridge, six
of them did it. One guy, unlike the embarrassed and
nauseated rest of them, got hooked. He kept huffing,
exhausting hours then days then seasons in those
fumes, until he could no longer navigate his way back
to the home he was raised in, or leave that home, or smile,
or speak as he lifted the

shot
gun

to
his
face

and

ble

w

it

clear

o
ff.

Diagnosis

A few years after high school, an old friend
was the first to diagnose me with I-thought-
you-were-going-to-be-something-
itis. A half-dozen Pils into our visit, he
candidly ventured, "a doctor, or a priest." I was
too stunned to reveal I really was something
mythic: a job-liberated, university-
disgorged, free time–trashing, mope-
robed Theseus, losing the labyrinth in a string
of antipodal successes. A Minotaur malformed
with the head of a man. My legs: the head of
a bull. Prescribed "cheer up," the chronic salvo
as salve for You're-just-down-in-the-
dumps-sclerosis, I never howled, "gloom
down," the legit call of all burrow-devoted, lice
nipped varmints, matted and aghast, addicted
to tunnels, the interred sun — our
dreams teeming with hundreds of hovel-sundered
beasts, scheming a meeting of horror and bottomless
love. To those who terminaled me with a case
of You're-such-a-loser-ismus, I should've,
clapping, spasmed: "This isn't stumbling you
regard. It's what happens while careening through
two worlds at once. Imagine that: one foot sopped in
earth, one foot out of time. I'm dancing, humming
with the music of all that's wrong, a melody

i
can
t

dis
robe

with
vo

ice

to
dre
ss

you
r

ear

Yesmads

How do
you herd the hordes of
eschatonal voices, the wound-
flocked visions? How do you caravan
their grunts, bays, and roars into
madrigal tunes? How do you pasture
in seasons of wrath? Forage in
flames? Produce proof when many claim
your hand's unburned, your mouth
unharmed? How do you roam
your cratered days and dare
to tell the truth of your travels? How
do you know who to trust with
the tale, having lived to tell
it? How do you keep living to
myth it? How do you tell while
tolled? Gather while hunted? Home
while haunted? Inscribe
as erased? How do you shelter,
unsettled, the strength to cry out

y
es

mad

you

are

my
t
ribe

MAD
MEN

The End Is in the Middle

Everyone at the airport is mad. A month into
"The Donald's" presidency, we're smiled into an elephantine line
and kept from departing Pearson. Beginning at US Customs,
our line stretches the length of Terminal 1, runs out of room, and
then forms a grumbling spiral in a shuttered check-in area, the end
buried in our swirling centre. Each new arrival exasperates, "Where
is the end?" Our mass refrains: "In the middle!" "Where?" "In
the middle!" we chorus again, and again. Authorities author our line
into this whorl. Power revises travel into tripping over luggage
until we bow, forcing us to learn force's motto, "the end is in
the middle," and to live, in this stymied line, its lesson, "the end
is here." Yet bound in the hold of this voyage-spoiling "middle,"
I do glimpse the shores of a very different significance. Doesn't
this dictum, repeated, give out tickets to its terminus, hinting that
this middle and its end can end? Doesn't its constriction strengthen
one's revolving to resolve the most open globe? To, resisting, scribe
riotous itineraries and elicit nourished pathways for all? To origin
destinations and lose the maps that hide each pilfered home? To
join the line we form to halt this command through its chanting,

"The

      end

  is

  in

the
    middle,"

  then
  be
  gin

Mine

Cure all your
hollow-boned friends, sick
with flight, ill with a tunnel
vision hell-bent on warning. Soak
their beacon-yellow feathers in
deeper shades of storm. Suffocate
their lungs with seed, certain
they must never sprout their song —
it's a reverse siren urging you away
from the rocky coasts you crave.
Remember, what you tear
from their mantles are not
wings but manacles. Don't
let their fluttering, finished, cage
your hunts. Pick their bones clean,
and on each carcass engrave
your warning to whatever follows:
"Kill the canaries before they can
die." Dig

your

tunnel

deeper
certain

it's

not

your
grave

Spring

It's the first day of spring training, when the osprey
flies its plump catch over the diamond and, after
landing in the oak behind left field, devours its
redfish feast. Below, before the anthems, we all
hold a moment of silence for the seventeen victims of
the Stoneman Douglas High shooting and for the two-
seam-fastball-hurling pitcher who crashed his plane
in the sea. The mismatch of these memorials is
outsized as the competitive gap between the talon-
weaponed raptor and the unarmed fish. The Jays and
Phils play united, wearing the same promotional ball
caps logoed with an *S*-hooked *D* in the
name of honouring memories. This is
the first step to forgetting. To remember,
finally, crest the bodies of the slaughtered
above the brim, replace the sharp, feeding breach
of osprey beak with a barrel. Some bro a row back
muses, "He had a great arm." Who did? The dead
pitcher? The living killer? Shakespeare hit a
homer of a line about this very moment: a ruler takes lives
as the osprey takes the fish — "by sovereignty of
nature." If only our nature was not this spring
training, practicing with bouncing bump stocks — no
safety — to get more out. If only our season had not
yet reached its opening day. Imagine if all our
centuries of hits, strikes, and driving lines into dirt
were really our training for our first, true spring, and

after

all

the
se

outs
we

ca
n

finally
reach

home

safe

Ballad of the Mad Bomber

A bomb is not a story, though
              Metesky claims to soothe
with rumour-spurring, blast-fed tales,
throning the search for truth.

          Through telephone and movie seat
      and subway coined with bombs,
George liens the wrongs and dastard debit
      yet owes each flame-scorched palm.

Sedate a dream with waking then
                rebrand each corpse a calf.
Explore "Mad Bomber"–planted visions,
          just slice your eyes in half.

      Though George elates he never killed,
designed his bombs to goad,
              if terror's free of fuse and charge

the

thr

eat

it

Se
lf.
Explo

des

Hope
Obama speech erasure poem

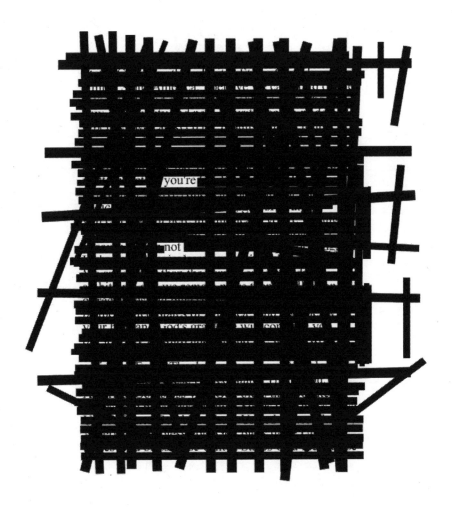

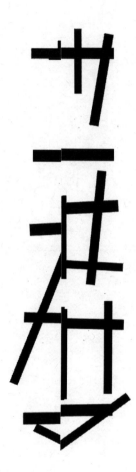

Imagination

Daniel can't imagine why he visits the Aurora theatre
where it happened. Maybe he's paying his respects
to the twelve, murdered doing what he loves most but
never imagined being killed doing. Maybe he's
battling the blasts of the villainous inner voice that
imagines him into a pyromantic duo with Holmes:
one rogue's blazing hate fevering for self-immolation
while the other just wants to watch the world burn.
Maybe in this night's rise, he fathoms how fancy's light
falls dark, caverns into a conceiving murk that is the
imagination's very own, a grim projector that blockbusters
the torturer's awakening of the political agitator
with a bed frame and car battery, origins the zealot's
faith-impelled van as urbane, cleansing round. Maybe
he's embarrassed for believing the imagination picks
sides, ashamed he didn't know its kryptonite is
the incapacity to make real a hero who can end its hells.
Maybe the remedy isn't catching a flick rife with
toy-hawking avengers who quip, "You get killed,
walk it off." Maybe if the memorial improvised
across the street for the victims had not been lost
to fresh construction, he would've remained in the
open light of the afternoon, honouring them through
a superpower everyone could share: hushed
attention. Or maybe the construction is the new
memorial, endlessly earth-moving excavators
and loaders rumbling as the truest monument for

whe

n

imagin

ation

fal

ters

or

fai

ls.

to

st

op

Refrain

Never again. N
ever again. Ne
ver again. Nev
er again. Neve
r again. Never
again. Never a
gain. Never ag
ain. Never aga
in. Never agai
n. Never again.
Never again. N
ever again. Ne
ver again. Nev
er again. Neve
r again. Never
again. Never a
gain. Never ag
ain. Never aga
in. Never agai
n. Never again.
Never again. N
ever again. Ne
ver again. Nev
er again. Neve
r again. Never
again. Never a
gain. Never ag
ain. Never aga
in. Never agai
n. Never again.

v

e

e

r

g

a

i

n.

Snowflake

                                    With gravity
                         and glee, I'm a snowflake who
                      teaches snowflakes to
                  uniquely blizzard with
                      snowflakes of words. Every myth,
                  at its most elemental, is a snowflake —
                      tongue-bound, avalanche
                          seed. I teach snowflakes, before
                  reading aloud, to say, CW, content
                      warning, for flurries, visibility, a cold
                  only snowflakes can carry from sky to
                  earth. I teach snowflakes CW, creative
                          warning, contently written forecasts
                  naming our blanket snowflake
                          truth: it's *because* we will melt
                          that we don't fear the light. Every
                          snowflake, at its most mythic, is an
                  oddity and amassed, a crystal
                          and the drift. You know you're
                          a snowflake if you don't find this
                  wonder abominable. If you find it
                      abominable, you've forgotten

y
o

u

a

r

e

s

n

o

w

Haiku

What if storm's force is
a flower's core? Petals, storm's
truth?

What
a flower

MAD
MAKING

Stops

A decade ago, I stepped to the edge of a subway
stop's platform. Something in me insisted a savage
stop: a track that loops "halt" mixed with "go," "jump
now," "end." The TTC stops short of calling these leaps
"suicides," settling on "personal injury at track level." Two
years ago, a jumper stopped all eastbound trains. The grove
of snapped vessels and bones the TTC's euphemism
branched through crackling speakers did not stop
commuters from raging in our train as we were
directed to exit. Angered, I called for respect, "stop
it," until an old woman stopped me, catching my eye
and arm in a way that said she had felt the push of
those unstoppable palms. Above ground, the slo-mo
murmuration of commuters resembled a vast knot of hair
stopping a drain. Those of us stuck with tickets to
this terminal — the leap, the swallow, the slice,
the blast — are tracked by this haunting, hunting
destination. Its muzzle tunnels into us visions of
that moment we finally arrive, its claws protract to cut
another record groove to loop its howl: "stop, stop,
stop." Shrinking, we whimper for a whiff of that fainter call
that echoes yet opposes this wail. It rises in the voice
of the man sitting beside me on the train, sparks this
poem. As I whisper my words into lines, he whispers
prayers from a book I can't place in a language I don't know
but somehow instantly grasp. The murmured chime of
his syllables mingle with my scribbles to hush
the trumpeting urge to end, soothing

stop
stop

stop

stop

stop

stop

now

Make

Why bother writing a poem? The future,
breaking away, doesn't want it. Even if
your lines are a monument to their moment,
tomorrow's fools will legislate new rules and
blast your statue, or extinct themselves into
stillness, the levelling left to sand and time. The
present's no different. Your poem may erect
a sustaining abode, but this home, at
best, ends up backgrounding a blockbuster scene
shared by the comic-book villain and his city-
obliterating bursts. And the past? Forget
it. Compose a time-travelling lyric that can
explore ancient centuries and it'll catch
a lethal influenza, its immunity lost, or it'll sustain
no senses or souls with its vision. If only poems
didn't need to be monuments and homes and
heroes. If only poems were seeds. It's no crisis
that most crack, rot, or blow away, the forest
made and remade over centuries through
the germinating few. If only poets were
the mythological creatures we never knew
— part skin, part song, part failed reach
and nailed loss. If only writing poems was
the same as making bread, the same workaday
labour, or the same as bread itself, a practice
that can

break

and

still

be
shared

can

sustain

and
is

made

new
each

day

Trials

Back in those days, none of my
stupidly excessive ingestions were attempts to
die; they were experiments undertaken to
substantiate poetry's power in my bodily life.

The twenty-six of tequila, tipped back in
two hours, arranged skin-tingling rhythms before
orchestrating retching's alliterative ruptures.

Blotters of acid and baggies of dried shrooms
ringed senses in imagery's vital veracity, each glimpse
ingrained with this truth: every thing knows everything.

This constricting fixed form — six amitriptyline with a side
of vodka — snared speech in one rule: "repeat
only the silence of the earth you black out on." Flesh's

Paxil-inspired cutting possessed metaphor's transformative
sorcery — my skin a door, blood a coast, skeleton a
sage who urges, "slice until the air breathes lung."

Today, my excess is writing, though none of these
lines scribbled, scratched out, replaced and refined,
fed ink and fruition starved, are attempts at poems;
they are

stu
die
s

in

B
ring
ing

de
at
h's

Pa
s
sage

To
li
fe

In the Fold

Daniel doesn't know what to do next. Rimple into
another illegally streamed cinematic disaster, Lethe
wallowing tower-defence game, or box of trans-fat–
themed cookies? Collapse concord in the world coiled
round his basement apartment? Enfold deeper in
the doughy layers of fusty blankets, subterranean gloom
re-baking his ache? He has not slept for days,
plenituding junk consumption. He has not *not* slept,
either. Time pleats, bunching him up with that semester he
shed waking and eating, dropped to one-forty, crumpling up
with tomorrow, his relief-devouring depression in
retreat but moaning in the cut, eager to zombie pounce
on gyrus and sulcus and feed. Sick-crinkled sediment
planted in the furrow of laptop and mattress, he germinates
like a fetus in a Murphy bed folded

into
the
wall
the
ro
om
re
pleni

shed
with
ce
ment

A ▶ ◀ B

If all we are
is form, then folds define
the simplest fury of our clipped
momentum, and all life is made possible
by folding in, by folding out. God
is the unfolding of disbelief's failure
to outwit the demand for the infinity
of a larger voice enfolded in bunches of a more
fragile breathing. Death is felt as the folding of
nothing into the paths the present ploughs under,
enclosures surrendered to enclosures, like mind
as the first model of incarceration, opening
up the possibility of sketching profiles of
tortured mobility and the belief that the moon
is some crazed fire ripped from the sky
on a moonless night and stuffed down
the throat of every enemy — until their
only and irreverent gift to the world is the least
tangible example of silence for the far-reaching
force of the speaking few. Love is the faintest feats
of hate folding tight around an impossible
adoration of distance. Hate
is love folding away from the hope
for some truncated distance, like a poem
as the folding-in fingers which, in closing,
escape their fisty fixity and dissolve into the briefest
palm. A poem

is
the
possible

infinity
of

enclosures
opening

on
their
only

impossible

escape

Upper Air Substance

All the experiences that stir my passion for alcohol are spirits
voyaging inside its names. Sipping, I summon ethyl's
                    Greek root; each drink erects a wanded, giddy lattice
                    I ascend to the "upper air substance" of inebriation, that
clumsily mixed cocktail of hot-faced hilarity and hug-
plunking love. The powdered antimony of the Arabic
                    al-kuhl is an eye-beclouding cosmetic that merges
          looking with shadow, beauty, smoke, and God, booze
               painting a celestial glow, the world muddled gorgeous.
The etymology of antimony pours me into a chair at
          the bar, ordering more, whether its meaning is squeezed from
          hypothetical Greek, *antimonos*, "against aloneness," or
dutifully shaken from real Greek, *antimonachos*, "monk killer,"
               a moniker concocted for alchemists poisoned in honest
               quests for gold. This source twists with the weird *cogito*
of crapulence, the antinomy of drinking: I'm juiced —
starkly powered and sapped, revived and drowned,
               a face applied to maelstrom, I mean, makeup,

A
vo
ice
that

plun
ges

from

du
st
to

star

Folderol

It's fitting — this remedy's alias sounds like a brand
of prescription drug. Chantix, Lunesta,
Concerta. Paxil, Prozac, Zoloft. Folderol: a treatment
tactile (pen, page, word) and intangible (word, spirit,
vision). Write poem after flimsy poem. Guaranteed
to cut down the meaningless refrains of your
symptoms — husking flurries, plunging seeds — with the
sickle of each poem's meaningless refrain. Helps stem
the outbreaks of trashitis, of treasurnoma's coziness,
prescribed by the geegaw of being. Side effects may
include a stiff wrist, a trifling addiction, blinding
clouds of paper rising from the lines of fire you remit
to the fires lining you, tweaked neck, odd filenames.
If feelings of wildness and devastation persist,

Con
tact

your

sick
ness,
prescribe

it
names.

Method

Why one
and not the other? Why poem and not
hastily splattered canvas
or mime? Why bullet
and not pill or bridge? Are we destined,
born into our craft, as with
the elemental signs of our birth?
Are calling and called, like surgeries,
linked? The Achilles can't be reattached
through the pupil; catheters will never
stem an artery's gush. Are we soulmates —
each me and each method, Cupid-
stabbed lovers together forever? What if
shuffling, veiled and trained, into this wedding
we're wrong? Maybe
the poem trying to ease pain is a wild mare
neighing a buzzsaw's wail. Maybe a bullet
sundering the skull is

a
h

and
with

A

stem

stabb
ing

the

sun

Don

Don Coles died today. Today, Katie,
a student I taught, published her first
                    book. I think of my teacher, Mike, who Don
                        taught, and I think of all the lessons that
            Don must have taught me through Mike, all
        Mike taught Katie through me. I think of
        the thirsty — cupped hands passing water into
                    cupped hands passing this water, without
breaks, into another cupped pair. I'm amazed
            at how much we can drink and still have more
    to share. I think of all I learned from Katie
                    just now, reading in the dusky subway light
                the first poem in her first book, and I am
            amazed at how the rapids of her lesson
    rush back through me to Mike to Don,
another tributary in this miracle river
                        that flows in both directions at once. It dawns
            on me how amazing it is that I'm a river
    at the same time that I'm a man underground,
breaking down on a train, at the same time
                that I'm a ceaseless pen, that I'm blurred words
            clarified through tears, that I'm ink that dreams
        it's

a
Don
that

breaks

to
light

another
dawns

breaking

MAD
COMPANIONS

Chances

Me and
a hundred-plus students flock around Roethke's elegy for his student,
taken by a chance accident. After the mandatory "Will this be on
the final?" the discussion soars — and I take a chance, giving
a personal reply to a question about the end. Roethke, as a teacher,
loved his student, just as I, *neither father nor lover*, love them,
their effort and potential, their imagination and voice. Mid-sentence, I
chance upon memories of the students I have lost, the two who took
their own lives beating into my vision like the wings of pigeons forced
off the sidewalk. I don't stand a chance: my admission transforms
into a sobbing plea — "Get help if you need it" — a bawling promise —
"I will do whatever I can." By chance, a student not enrolled in this
class, attending with a friend who thought she'd like it, is caged by the
isolating need to take her life. By chance, I am in my office two nights after,
working late, when she knocks, asks if I have a second, and weeps
when I say yes. She is a stone owl trapped in a snow globe shaken by
her sickness, by her parents who deny she is ill, by the imam who
testifies she is possessed by the devil, by the relentless voice that
teaches her why, how, when (now) to end it. Listening is a miracle avian:
its song a seminar on singing, its flight a lesson on
taking flight. An hour in, I can see she glimpses it: feathers survive beneath
stone; the globe's glass, shattered, can give way to sky. No hold is
final. I've got a question for the final. The answer is way beyond
me, though I know its truth, above all others, must be studied and
shared. How do we nurture such chance intersections of our veering
migrations, where taking a chance gives a chance,

and

giving
a

chance

transforms

this

isolating

test
teaches
its
taking
is

shared.

Topé Suicida

Isled in the ring, foe tossed out,
the wrestler dives through
fight-framing ropes headfirst, skies
this death-hailing move.
Wrestlers can't risk necks
or fight for their art; their art

Is
the
fight
this death

MAD Fans

sung to the tune of Lorde's "Royals"

We've never seen a ruler *MAD* can't "Blech!"
We cut our teeth on skewerings of ads and movies
Like parodies of pop-song dreck
The self-absurding gag, we want truth humoured madly

'Cause every cover shows
Alfred E. Neuman gap-toothed and transforming
Usurping headlines, bearing history's moorings
What a deal
The cost might rise but the price stays "Cheap!"

Gawd, every issue's got
Snappy Jaffee, *MAD* Looks, Martin's sproinging
Sergioed margins, Jacked stars, spies purloining
What a steal
This cracked Proteus of magazines

And we'll always be *MAD* fans (*MAD* fans)
Applauding each timely spoof
Id-inking putzes are for us
We crave schmuck-scripted laugh riots
Let's holler we're fools, here (fools, here)
Exclaiming we are proudly mad
'Cause, Fonebone, we're fools,
We're fools, we're fools, we're fools

Like
The

Usu
al

Ga
ng

of
Id
iots

Napkin

Daniel doesn't know that a party is a camera. He almost
cancels his fortieth because of the stigmata of mental
illness. A party hands us an animated album of ourselves,
outside and in: cinema meets inhalation meets cardiogram
meets doodle. His sickness, he believes, is visible as
wounds, weeping and grisly; they'll scare everyone off,
spoil the dip, or attract incredulous fingers, earthy
digits probing his alien pain. A party is a bouquet of
reminders we are worthy of life and love. Daniel can
never say this: "I'm worthy of such and such." He dreads
the whole gang's coming over to reveal he's the miracle
sore erupting on a sentient gash. Instead, his
friends arrive, embrace him, and the party is ravioli
meets midsummer: a fresh-sun aromaed, verdancy-stuffed
feast. In the morning, tidying up, he's a gleaner, the party's
garbage his harvest. The sour empties, cake-peppered
plates, sticky mystery spills, canthi of cigarette butts, and
the landed sky lanterns of crumpled napkins souvenir
the party's ebullient album: collage meets kaleidoscope
meets calliope meets cascade. In memory's revelry,
he mistakes a gift for garbage. It's not a napkin but
a homemade card he saves from the trash, a present
from a best bud's little boy. For "Danio," the friend
had said in loving imitation of his son, identifying the
looping crayon lines as horses. Though Danio still
does not see the horses, he does feel himself riding
one, feels the night wind's crisp snap, the striding
gale of the horse slowing as they round a hill's curve
and he glimpses a light up ahead, a fire labouring
in the dark, the flickering of the people who built it —
and shaking the reins, quickening that gale, he hollers,
like a wild "yee-haw,"

i

am

wo

rthy

of

li

fe

and

lo

ve

Hope

I ask friends for help
writing a poem about hope
and Nehal asks, "Isn't hope the most
devastating device?" The "tin
windup duck on a trike," Catriona
describes, "pedalling while its hat
propeller twirls, hallucinating
flight." Or whatever contrivance
devised the "clear-cut forest" Ted says
"the people wake up to" — "trash trees
grow first, tall and fast. Die and feed."
Hope, for Brian, "cradles"; is, for Safa,
"necessary to cope"; "weaves
tapestries of dreams," for Grayson,
"blankets against doubt." Zahra soars
hope as the "butterflies that can't migrate;
I cough them up and set them free." But
where? Into Mattieu's "silence that
sneaks into the sizzling air"? Into Jeff's "rain that
moves downwards upwards
all at once" and
"in the indecision
once again I can"? Hopeful,
always, Oubah lunars, "we
trace a new moon over
that empty expanse," while Jim, too, cultivates
a clearing, beginning, "hope fills
the hollow between two…," and then
leaves the line unfinished for our words,
hopeful as

ope

n

flight

gro

ves

,

oars

that

move
all

,
a
trace
that
fills

War on Terror

I let my sister down as poems
     composed to protest Bush's bombs
letter the café's gallant hush.
      This stranger, sister, mutters. Shushed,
   she shouts, then shouts fire back scorched alms.

I don't dissent, ignore the psalms,
mythic with terror, illness homes
 silently in soul and flesh,
   and, silent, let my sister down.

Sternly, poets help spread calm,
 dousing her strife with forced aplomb:
   "Please, leave!" We're healed through hurts we crush.
We do not free our ears to gush
 new pools of care into whose balm

I

let

my
si

Ster
do

W
n

Mad Lib

We demand
the right to [Verb 1]
[Noun 1]s, the freedom to, arising,
[Adverb] call them
[Adjective 1] [Noun 2]s,
to [Verb 2] them
like banished
[Noun 3]s. We demand
licence to [Verb 3]
the [Adjective 2] night,
the sovereignty to [Verb 4]
the [Noun 4] as our
[Adjective 3] cure.
Liberated, we are mad
as [Noun 5]s, nuts as
the [Noun 6]s that [Verb 5]
into the very
heart of the [Adjective 4]
[Noun 7], into the fire of
[Adjective 5] [Noun 8]s.
Mad, we are liberated
as the

[Noun 1]
        hem

        m
        ed

        li
        ght,

the

Li

        very

        of
[Noun 8]s.

Bi-Lungual

The lungs of our
dead fold into our lungs like a letter
into an envelope, a wick into a
candle's flame. Inhaling, we
fill the lobes that nourished their
words, heaving the dim, urgent
breadth of their flickering.

The lungs of our
dead enfold ours like the
forge embraces iron, a quickening
blaze. Even as we suffocate
(our bronchi idle, each alveolus
stuffed with numb),

our

dead

can

brea

the

for

us

The Middle Is in the End

I love how nothing will survive in these lines
to you, love. They will, over time, mature into
mirrors in a world without reflections. Like all
lines, eventually, they will die. I love that we
will die. The blanket your life wraps around
my life will unravel. The warping my life
blankets your life in will tatter and vanish along
with the bed we tangled, our room, our sleep
ceasing its drift in this sleep. It's a dream — to
have survived long enough to reach this end. What
a prize. This dream. This death. The middle is
in the end: the viscera of our meeting, the nerves
of our intimate endurance, the blastulas of our
ecstasies sustain and sense and conceive our deaths'
unbeating, banded hearts. Without you, I never
could have blossomed an autumn body's
wintery after. This is how thankful
snow must feel falling, blessed with a cradling
earth to blanket. The joy earth bursts, graced
by time with space to form. Space's elation
as it expands, voiding nothing. How amazing
to have had the chance to expand and form
and fall with you, like snow drifting beyond its dock
into melting, like a planet, evaporated, unhinging
from wholeness, the cosmos conceding to

MORE
MAD
ME

Sonnet

My sickness grips like origami crossed
　　　　with drowning — folding forms that flood. My neck's
a sinking crane. My nerves are stars wave tossed,
　　my mind a paper boat that ebbs and wrecks.
Handled like salt by tongue, a mutt that's told
　to die, I play at death and brawl to not
　　　　　dissolve, but in this clash I twist and hold,
　I bend and keep the new creased forms sick wrought.
　　　　That's why I need its craft. Its folds — missing
then offed — would match a lover's failing joist,
drink down to dust all teachers' wells, abyssing
　　the heights of words and lifting depths from voice.
　　So to this grip that drives my throat to sink,

My
neck's
a

Hand
to
hold,
I
sing
then
drink

Dead Cemetery

The underworld of Kerouac's praise for madness: that
which drives one to be mad to live and talk can be that which
one desires with each mad breath and word to kill. It's
dwelled in me from the start, one of my earliest memories, it
and its lesson that it will never leave, that it will never stay
still or shushed or driven into shovel-scoured earth with bone
breaking force — the it that is I, the self I wish could be
morgued and buried in a cemetery that dies, the worst self
entrailed in the self right from the start, the self our best
self is buried in the soil of, and all our ways of dealing
are failures to claw through the dirt to the light with two
broken hands. The petrified squirm of this outward
inward dig uncovers the arithmetic of addiction,
the addition of subtraction, subtraction by addition —
drinking and writing. Filling these incalculable
notebooks — this page, right now — is like drinking,
a mystifying mix of escape and connection, of division
and immersion, the melody of one harmonizing with the
other sublimely: just one more sip, just one more
word, just one more shot, just one more page, just
one more night like this and I'll exceed it, just one
more work written finally just right at last and I'll say
exactly what it is I need to erase, the moment Kerouac
invoked before he burned out, the ash end of a Roman
candle dashed in the gutter-gathered rain, "One day
I will find the right words, and they will be simple." Until

that

one
d
ay
one

mor
e

wo
rd

the

n

an
other

o
more

Bad Hand

A "bad hand" is what we call disasters to shuffle
    a little hope into job loss, illness, divorce — tragedy
                as a hand we can fold to wait for winning
                  cards. But the bad hand
    of this voice is so ingrained, it's like the cards are
    stitched to my fingers. This voice's hate, in turn, grips
        me like I'm the bad hand it flopped right after, possessed
by a gut feeling, betting everything. How does
    a hand fold its holder? What features beyond this
      detaining player must it muck to win: the table's
            other shuffling schlubs, the room, the game
    itself? And what if one of us did it — collapsed the deck-
thatched house? We don't. Instead, we hold. This voice
yearns for new profanities to bark at its cards, wishing,
        like the king of hearts, I'd drive a sword deep into
    my crown. I invent new figures for the cards stitched
    to my palms. They're a fan, feathers, a mask to
disappear behind as I play at hoping, no, betting, I'm

A

winning
hand

possessed
by
a

game

that
yearns
to

disappear

Psycho Sometimes

"We all just go a little mad sometimes."
What Norman claims for all is true of horror.
Though horror shows the mad with knives in grime,
do film's raw manias exhibit more?

Though Norman's claim for all is true of horror,
with sickness masked in vengeful violent splats,
film's grotesque manias might offer more
than kills repeating kills, illness begat.

This sickness, masked in vengeful violent splats,
projects onscreen what gnaws my insides, feasts.
Look, films repeating kills, illness begat,
snap gingerly with frames my sickening beast.

Project on screens what gnaws my guts and skin —
this feeds a diagnosis game. I beam,
"I'm sick with *Ginger Snaps*, *The Beast Within*,
a case of *Psycho*, *Nightmare* spells. I'm *Scream*ed."

Horror feeds a hopeful aim: in steam,
shower-bound, the final girl, I strive
to face my psycho nightmare spells and scream,
"Horror, against my horrors you urge, 'Survive!'"

Shower-bound, the final girl, I thrive.
A little mad most times, I'll always go
with horror versus horror to survive.
For knived or grimed,

at.

L
east.

this

Horror
show

S

Major Depressive Disorder
DSM-5 *found poem*

Sadness may be denied
at first, inferred from
facial expression and demeanor. The individual
          looks as if he or she is about to cry. Sadness may be
denied. Feeling "blah," having no feelings, or feeling anxious,
          a depressed mood can be inferred from the person's facial expression
                    and demeanor, described by
          the person as depressed, sad, hopeless,
               discouraged, or "down in the dumps," an
          intense wish to end what is perceived as an unending
and excruciatingly painful emotional state. They have to
force themselves to eat. Some individuals emphasize
somatic complaints, report or exhibit increased irritability,
     feeling less interested in hobbies, "not caring anymore,"
or not feeling any enjoyment, an inability to foresee any
enjoyment in life (a formerly avid golfer no longer plays,
          a child who used to enjoy soccer finds excuses not
               to practice). A person may report sustained fatigue without
     physical exertion, complain that washing and dressing
in the morning are exhausting and take twice as long
as usual, misinterpret neutral or trivial day-to-day events as
evidence of personal defects and have an exaggerated
sense of responsibility for being sick and for failing. Many
          individuals report impaired ability to think, concentrate,
               or make even minor decisions, complain of memory
          difficulties, wish to not be a burden to others, a passive wish
not to awaken in the morning, or a belief that others
would be better off if the individual were

a
fac
e
denied
expression
scribed by

an
ending

without

evidence
sense

memory
wish

Eurydicinema

Daniel doesn't know he will never grow out of it. Alone in
the film school's basement, he's a mature student, editing
              a short that explores the cinema as Orpheus. Debilitated
grub transforming into healed beetle — that's how he pictures cutting
depression. Maturing, age halting madness's reeling. The cured unbound
              and beautiful, husking the cocoon. He's got it all wrong.
                        Eurydice's is the truer story. The earth closing above her opens
up the underworld, frees her from the same old shrouding
              singer, cloaking tune. Not — presto! — wings, but lobster's
andante moulting composes the metamorphosis of Daniel's illness,
shedding one rigid, homely skin for another. Thank the gods
              for Eurydice. Pioneer of perdition. Hell guide. She weathers nether-
realm tunnels, clashes with spectres and monsters, digs away
                        skeletoned roots, surfaces to save fragments of light on torches
              original and familiar, inventing cinema, reanimating song.
Out of anywhere, at any age, depression returns. It's the unkillable
                        B-movie creature turned filmmaker. The slasher-flick butcher
as editor, cutting, splicing, making *Tiz*, a trash film, worse. The
hack writer scribbling him as gruesome superhero: skinned,
              nerves bared like a scared dog's chompers, his hide like
              a blindfold tied over his eyes, a misplaced cape. Even though
              Eurydice's myth did not survive, except in its absence, look
      down —

the

gr
   ound

   opens
up

and
she

rea
   ches

Out
   her

ha
n

d

We Are

We are, rare prisoners, sentenced to escape.
This skill to flee our urge to die's our cage.
We're rocket ships that veer off course to snake
    through vacuumed void or ink a planet's page
with crashing crafts: we slip the graves that lake
below our skin and wade in streams that stage

    evading paths but end as waterfalls.
Take me, eighteen, eluding suicide
    through fevered gulps of poems and alcohol —
above my bed tape Clare's "I Am," inside
young thirst plunge vodka shots, re-read, re-pour.
My death's the chow that words and drink devour.

    I long to still my drive to halt, attend,
with soil, to grain sky-reared by savage weather,
this loam emerging where our struggles blend,
evincing what we are we are together.
Like now, I'm cloth unfurled, you're vibrant dye,

This

    page

below

    —

above
  you
    r.

    tend,
    er,

  e
    ye,

Gift

Mom bought me my very first issue of
MAD magazine when I was six. It was a gift I forced,
keenly sneaking the Alfred E. Neuman-as-gremlin cover onto
the checkout at Seve. Each month after, engrossed on sofa
or bus or lawn, I was committed to the gift of a new issue, an axil
of wildness from which stemmed leaves of wonder and glee.
Many akin gifts were stacked with this one: the hull of a home
keeled by books, the newsprint roll Dad expanded in the kitchen
for us to co-draw space wars, the toy guns we aimed at the alfalfa
in search of hiding spies, the Olivetti I "hunted and pecked" to coil
the veins of stories onto paper's blank brain, movie night
lighting any night, the journals for hiving verse's honey
and sting. Of all the gifts my parent shared, the one I save
lifelong for how it saved my life, the gift that like an atmosphere
contains and sustains the rest, is the perpetually posted missive
lettered by their love: "It's okay to fail," a stocking stuffed with
lingual treats — "stay wild," "go mad," "gremlin perfection," "trip
into slipping's lift." Even opened, this present stays packaged
to give again, words to receive, unwrap within, and revive:

MA
ke
fa
il

Ma
ke
fa
il

li
ve
li
ve
l

ive:

A Mad Fold-In Poem

You — this mucky fire slathered in my mind's frame
— are as committed to me as artists are to art. At times,
your voice is constant: "Kill yourself, kill yourself, kill
yourself" — fists punching clay with the aim to make me
nothing more than punched clay. Other times, you're
a cinema in my skull, screening me mangled: leg
auger-mauled, hand vice-crushed, eye pencil-blinded to
life. "End it," you say, in the scene you loop: this cinema's walls
with a bullet burst. At parties, you shape a sinister play from
others' glances: "hate him," "idiot," "fool." When I bloom,
a sun, all alight and rising, you flatten my lift into lines
on a page like Jaffee's in the back of *MAD*. You fold it
over and now the rise is the wound from a wing cleaved
and then gilded, the bloom's a thousand-foot fall, the sun
a drain. Yet with each step the unrelenting chorus of you
circles round me, another chorus surfaces to surround you: the
line of sheltering trees artists grow, loamy and ablaze, against
your gale, the melodies of friends whose works asphyxiate your
symphony, the lessons students teach about tipping your
plinths, the magic of bringing nib to page and penning life
with urgency and patience, word by word, with abandon
and care. Even though I know it can never silence you, I love
this inky trick because it fills the blank before you can, marks
up your script, swallows you choking in a page-mutating
fold, so your cruel barks, garbled, almost seem to say:

frame

your

life
with
others'
lines

and
you

line
your

life
with
love

Notes

The sources of the epigraphs are poker pro Stu "The Comeback Kid" Ungar and professional wrestler Eddie "The Mad King" Kingston.

"Our Kind" is written, with gratitude, for Anne Sexton.

The text for the erasure poem "Hope" is Barack Obama's re-election speech.

"Topé Suicida" is a fold-in seguidilla. A topé suicida (Spanish for "suicide head-butt") is a professional wrestling move. It involves the wrestler diving headfirst through the ropes at an opponent outside the ring.

"Hope" is a collaborative fold-in poem. Thank you to the following dear poet friends for your generous contributions: Grayson Chong, Nehal El-Hadi, Brian Guan, Jim Johnstone, Jeff Latosik, Safa Minhas, E Martin Nolan, Oubah Osman, Mattieu Ramsawak, Zahra Tootonsab, and Catriona Wright.

"War on Terror" is a fold-in rondeau.

"*Psycho* Sometimes" is a fold-in pantoum.

The text for the found poem "Major Depressive Disorder" is drawn from the "Diagnostic Features" portion of the "Major Depressive Disorder" section of the *DSM-5*.

"We Are" is written, with gratitude, for John Clare.

Acknowledgements

Thank you to all the talented and hardworking people at *Arc, Best Canadian Poetry, Carousel, CV2, diode, Grain, Long Con, OOMPH!, Poetry, Poetry Is Dead, Tampa Review,* the *Ampersand Review,* the *Fiddlehead, untethered,* and *White Wall Review* for publishing a selection of these poems. Thank you to Frog Hollow Press for producing the gorgeous 2021 chapbook, *Mad Fold-In Poems.*

Thank you to the judges and contest organizers who recognized some of the work contained here. "Folderol" was named runner-up for the *Puritan*'s Thomas Morton Prize. "Don" and "Spring" received Honourable Mention in the *New Quarterly*'s Nick Blatchford Occasional Verse Contest. "Lift" was longlisted for the *Fiddlehead*'s Ralph Gustafson Prize for Best Poem.

Thank you to the Canada Council and Sage Hill Writing for supporting the creation of this work.

Thank you to the brilliant friends whose advice, feedback, and contributions significantly improved the works in this collection. Thank you Geoff Bouvier, David James Brock, Brian Guan, Esau Hussain, Jim Johnstone, Ryanne Kap, Sylvia Legris, Nathan Mader, Téa Mutonji, Tolu Oloruntoba, SJ Sindu, Priscila Uppal, Vanessa Vigneswaramoorthy, and Andrew Westoll for your feedback and belief.

Thank you, Susanne, Alan, and Julie; the icehouse poetry board; Martin Ainsley, and James Langer.

Thank you, Richard Wang, for the glorious fold-in cover image and author's portrait. You have captured me in my favourite state: joyful and eager with just the right touch of "happy-go-lucky wiseacre" (of which Harvey Kurtzman would approve).

Thank you to all the students I teach, who I learn with and from. Thank you to my family, always. Always, thank you to Andrea Charise for loving, inspiring, and sustaining your mawd mawn.

Thank you to *MAD*, to the mad, and to this madness.

What, we worry?

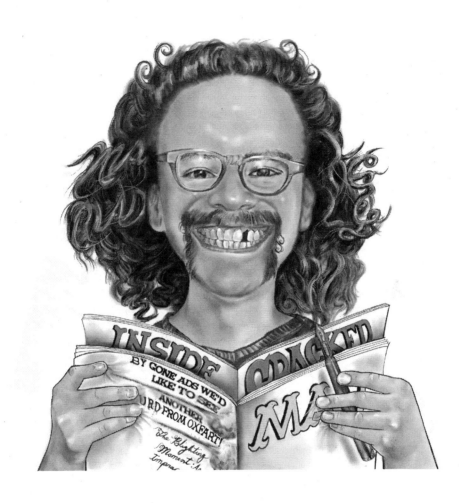

Daniel Scott Tysdal is a writer, filmmaker, and teacher. An Associate Professor, Teaching Stream, at the University of Toronto Scarborough, Tysdal's works include the ReLit Award-winning poetry collection *Predicting the Next Big Advertising Breakthrough Using a Potentially Dangerous Method*, the critically acclaimed *Fauxccassional Poems*, the short story collection *Wave Forms and Doom Scrolls*, the poetry textbook *The Writing Moment: A Practical Guide to Creating Poems*, and the viral TEDx talk, "Everything You Need to Write a Poem (and How It Can Save a Life)." Tysdal's short films have been screened internationally, earning him several honours, including Best Experimental Short Film at the Arizona Underground Film Festival, a nomination for Best Experimental Short Film at the Yorkton Film Festival, and the Intertoto Award at the Videodrunk Film Festival. *The End Is in the Middle* is his fourth collection of poetry.